100 Healthy Smoothies:

Healthy Smoothies for Optimal Health, Weight-Loss, Increased Energy, and Longevity

Sara Wilson

Table of Contents

Introduction

Congratulations on purchasing your personal copy of *100 Healthy Smoothies: Healthy Smoothies for Optimal Health, Weight-Loss, Increased Energy, and Longevity.* Thank you for doing so.

The following chapters will show you many ways you can enjoy a healthy smoothie using a few simple guidelines. Some of them include:

- Use whole fruit to provide fiber and reduce hunger pains.

- Don't skip the green veggies, they provide a nice coloring as well as healthy nutrients. Even if you don't like them in a salad, they are delicious as part of a smoothie.

- Be sure to provide some omega-3 fatty acids with a tablespoon of flaxseed meal.

- Consume some unsaturated fat such as a tablespoon of nut butter or half of an avocado.

- Provide plenty of ice for the smooth texture.

There are plenty of books on this subject on the market, thanks again for choosing this one! Every effort was made to ensure it is full of as much useful information as possible, please enjoy!

Chapter 1
#1 Smoothie – Blueberry Smoothies

As a quick note, you will notice throughout the steps provided for each smoothie, coconut cream is mentioned in some of them. In case you are new to the smoothie world, this is the thick creamy stuff found in the top of the can of full-fat coconut milk. Also, most of the products used for the smoothies are available at supermarkets such as Wal-Mart, so you don't have to stress whether you can purchase the necessary ingredients for the tasty drinks.

Please enjoy!

#1 Smoothie Worldwide

Ingredients

6 frozen strawberries

1 banana

1 cup plain non-fat yogurt

½ cup orange juice

Instructions

1. Combine the juice, banana, yogurt, and berries for 20 seconds using a high-speed blender.

2. Pause and scrape down the sides and blend 15 more seconds. Heaven!

Yields: One serving

Acai - Super Smoothie

Ingredients

2 bananas

1 package (3 ½ ounces) frozen acai puree – unsweetened

1 cup of each:

- Frozen raspberries

- Pomegranate juice

1 tablespoon agave nectar

Instructions

1. In a blender, add the acai puree and the remainder of the ingredients.

2. Process the smoothie using a high-speed blender until smooth.

Yields: 2 large drinks

Apple Pie Smoothie

Ingredients

1 medium apple

1 tsp. ground cinnamon

¼ tsp. each:

- Freshly ground nutmeg

- Ground cardamom

½ cup old-fashioned oats

1 tbsp. brown sugar

½ tsp. vanilla extract

1 ½ cups apple juice

Instructions

1. Program the oven temperature to 400°F.

2. Add some parchment paper to a small baking sheet.

3. Use a fork to mix the spices and brown sugar in a mixing dish. Toss in the slices of apple to evenly coat them. Arrange the sugared apples on the sheet and bake ten minutes.

4. Dump the oats on another sheet and remove them after five minutes.

5. Let both pans cool.

6. Pulse the oats in a blender until finely ground, and combine the remainder of the ingredients. Blend for approximately 30 seconds until smooth.

Yields: 1 serving (16 ounces)

Avocado Smoothie - Keto

Ingredients

6 drops –EZ-sweetz – or your brand sweetener

3 ounces unsweetened almond milk

1 avocado

3 ounces heavy whipping cream

6 ice cubes

Instructions

1. Slice the avocado into halves, remove the seeds and flesh, and toss it into the mixer along with the remainder of ingredients.

2. Add the ice and blend until creamy smooth.

Serving Portion: One serving

Avocado Smoothie - Regular

Ingredients

14 ounces full-fat milk

2 chopped frozen bananas

1 cubed avocado

Instructions

1. Combine everything in a blender and blend until well mixed. Enjoy!

Yields: Two servings

Avocado Blueberry Smoothie

Ingredients

1 cup almond milk

½ cup each:

- Baby romaine lettuce

- Frozen blueberries

¼ avocado – peeled and no pit

2 tablespoons dry old-fashioned oats

1-2 Medjool pitted dates

1 tablespoon raw sunflower seeds

½ teaspoon ground cinnamon

Instructions

1. Add all of the components into a high-speed blender. Go from the lowest to the highest setting in 35 seconds. Enjoy pronto!

Yields: One serving

Banana - Blueberry – Soy Smoothie

Ingredients

1 ¼-cups light soy milk

½ frozen sliced banana

½ cup frozen loose-pack blueberries

1 teaspoon pure vanilla extract

2 packages artificial sweetener/2 teaspoons sugar

Instructions

1. Pour one cup of the milk with the sweetener/sugar, banana, blueberries, and vanilla.

2. Blend until smooth using the highest speed, usually about 20 to 30 seconds.

Note: You can add up to ¼ cup of milk if you prefer a thinner smoothie.

Yields: Two servings

Banana – Cocoa Soy Smoothie

Ingredients

½ cup each

- Silken tofu

- Soy milk

1 tablespoon honey

1 banana

2 tablespoons unsweetened cocoa powder

Instructions

1. Cup up and freeze the banana.

2. In a blender, add the milk, cocoa, honey, and tofu – blend until smooth.

Note: Add the banana bits through the hole in the top (if there is one) with the motor running, and continue blending until creamy.

Yields: One serving

Banana Ginger Smoothie

Ingredients

¾ cup (6 ounces) vanilla yogurt

1 sliced banana

½ teaspoon freshly grated ginger

1 tablespoon honey

Instructions

1. Combine the banana, yogurt, honey, and ginger. Blend for about 30 seconds. Add a few ice cubes too if you wish.

Yields: Two servings

Banana Mint Smoothie

Ingredients

1/3 cup water

1 peeled – frozen banana

2 tablespoons each:

- Almond/peanut butter

- Cacao powder

Instructions

1. Add everything into the blender and combine until smooth.

Note: To create a different taste, add a handful of raw almonds, protein powder, 2 tablespoons of raw oats or unsweetened coconut. Also, add a pinch of ground cinnamon.

Yields: One serving

Banana Oatmeal Smoothie

Ingredients

½ cup low-fat plain yogurt

¼ cup old-fashioned rolled oats

½ cup almond milk

1 banana cut into thirds

¼ teaspoon ground cinnamon

Optional: 1 teaspoon honey

Instructions

1. Combine everything, blend about 30 seconds until mixed, and enjoy.

Yields: One serving

Basil – Kiwi Smoothie

Ingredients

1 cup plant milk (rice used)

½ cup each:

- Frozen cut leaf spinach

- Frozen mango chunks

4 leaves Italian basil

1 kiwi

1 pitted Medjool date

¼ cup raw almonds

Instructions

1. Peel and quarter the kiwi.

2. Combine all of the fixings to a blender using the high-speed setting for approximately 30 seconds. Enjoy immediately.

Yields: One serving

Berry Breakfast Smoothie

You can use the berries of your choice; such as blackberries, raspberries, strawberries, or blueberries.

Ingredients

1 ¼ cups each:

- Berries

- Orange juice

1/2 cup plain yogurt

1 banana

1 ¼- cup orange juice

Optional: 1 tablespoon Splenda® Granular

Instructions

1. Mix all of the fixings using a blender until your smoothie creamy. Serve right away.

Yields: Three servings (One cup each)

Blackcurrant Smoothie

Ingredients

¼ cup each:

- Coconut milk/heavy whipping cream

- Strawberries - fresh/frozen

½ cup each:

- Water

- Blackcurrants – frozen/fresh

½ vanilla bean or 1/2 teaspoon sugar-free vanilla extract

5-7 drops stevia extract/low-carb sweetener - optional

2 tablespoons chia seeds – whole or powdered

Instructions

1. Combine the milk/cream, berries, water, blackcurrants, vanilla, sweetener, and chia seeds in a blender. Pulse the ingredients until creamy smooth.

2. Let it set about two minutes and enjoy!

Yields: One serving

Blueberry – Coconut – Chia Smoothies

Ingredients

1 cup each:

- Full-fat Greek yogurt/almond milk/coconut milk

- Frozen blueberries

- Unsweetened almond/cashew milk

2 tablespoons each:

- Ground chia seed

- Coconut oil

Sweetener equivalent to 2 tablespoons sugar; your favorite

½ cup coconut cream

Optional: Protein powder or other supplements

Instructions

1. Mix everything together in a blender and enjoy!

Yields: Three to four servings

Blueberry Magic

Ingredients

½ cup unsweetened almond milk

¾ cup frozen blueberries

1 tablespoon almond butter

Instructions

1. Blend all three ingredients until smooth.

2. Consider the possibilities of 1 teaspoon pure vanilla extract, a frozen peeled banana, some fresh ginger, or 2 tablespoons of rolled oats or flax meal.

Yields: One serving

Blueberry Muffin Smoothie

Ingredients

½ cup unsweetened vanilla almond breeze/your choice

4-6 ounces vanilla Greek yogurt (individual size)

½ frozen/whole (for a sweeter smoothie) banana

½ cup frozen blueberries

¼ teaspoon lemon zest

¼ cup raw – uncooked- gluten-free oats

½ cup ice cubes

Instructions

1. Toss all of the goodies into a blender, adding the ice cubes last.

2. Blend for about two minutes until creamy smooth.

Yields: One serving

Blueberry – Peanut Butter Smoothie

Ingredients

1 cup ice cubes

¼ cup almond milk

2 tablespoons whey protein

½ cup frozen/fresh blueberries

1 tablespoon peanut butter

1 banana

Instructions

1. Mix it all in a high-speed blender for about 20-30 seconds, and enjoy!

Yields: One serving

Blueberry – Strawberry- Banana Smoothie

Ingredients

1 medium banana

1 cup skim milk

½ cup each:

- Blueberries

- Strawberries

Optional:

- Garnish: 1-2 fresh mint leaves

- 1 cup ice cubes

Instructions

1. Chop the banana and add the remainder of the ingredients to a blender.

2. Blend about 30 seconds and enjoy.

Yields: One serving

Chapter 2
Cherry - La Isla Bonita Smoothies

Cherry – Almond Smoothie

Ingredients

1 cup of each:

- Almond Breeze – Vanilla Almond Coconut Milk

- Fresh/frozen cherries

3 tbsp. raw almonds

2 tbsp. raw honey

1 tsp. cinnamon

½ tsp. almond extract

1 tbsp. coconut oil

Instructions

1. Using a blender, mix the milk, cherries, honey, almond extract, and cinnamon.

2. Add ice if you use fresh cherries, and process until smooth.

3. Dump the coconut oil into the blender while it's in operation.

4. Fill your glass with the tasty treat, and sprinkle with some cinnamon.

Yields: One serving

Cherry – Kiwi Smoothie

Ingredients

1 kiwi

1 cup of each:

- Frozen cherries

- Almond milk

1 tablespoon chia seeds

Instructions

1. Peel and chop the kiwi – reserving two slices for garnish. Add them to the blender.

2. Toss in all of the tasty goodies, blending until smooth.

3. Garnish with a couple of kiwi slices.

Cherry – Peach Smoothie

Ingredients

6 ounces black cherry/peach Chobani Greek Yogurt

1 fresh peach/or 1 cup frozen slices

1 cup fresh/frozen sweet cherries

1-2 cups fresh/frozen baby spinach

¼ - ½ cup milk – unsweetened vanilla almond was used – your choice

Instructions

1. Combine the peaches, cherries, and yogurt in a blender, and add the spinach.

2. Add ¼ cup of the milk and blend until smooth. Add the other ¼ cup if you want it thinner.

Yields: One serving

Cherry – Vanilla – Green Smoothie

Ingredients

1 medium banana

2 cups dark sweet frozen cherries

1 tablespoon ground flaxseed

½ teaspoon pure vanilla extract

2 cups unsweetened coconut milk

1 cup kale

Note: Water for consistency

Instructions

1. Place each ingredient into a blender, adding water if needed.

2. Process the smoothie until creamy.

Yields: Two servings

Chia Blueberry Coconut Smoothie

Ingredients

1 cup full-fat Greek yogurt/coconut or almond milk for vegan – dairy free

1 cup frozen blueberries

½ cup coconut cream

1 cup almond or cashew milk - unsweetened

2 tablespoons each:

- Ground chia seed

- Coconut oil

Sweetener equivalent 2 tablespoons sugar

Optional: Protein powder/or another supplement

Instructions

1. Blend until all ingredients are smooth. Pour into four glasses and enjoy.

Yields: Four servings (Keto)

Chocolate Avocado Raspberry Smoothie - Keto

Ingredients

1 ¼-cup Silk Cashew Milk

1/3 cup frozen raspberries

½ avocado

1 tablespoon cocoa powder

1/8 teaspoon raspberry extract

Sweetener to Taste: 1 tablespoon powdered Swerve – what I used

Instructions

1. Add it all to the blender, but for a thinner smoothie, add another ¼ cup of the cashew milk.

Yields: Two servings

Chocolate - Banana - Almond Butter Smoothie

Ingredients

1 frozen banana

1 cup almond milk - unsweetened

1 tablespoon each:

- Almond butter

- Homemade fat-free chocolate syrup

1 handful of ice

Ingredients for the Syrup:

1 ½ cup each:

- Organic sugar

- Water

1 teaspoon vanilla extract

1/8 teaspoon salt

1 cup cocoa powder

Instructions

1. *For the syrup*: Bring the ingredients (omit the vanilla) to a boil in a medium saucepan. Pour in the vanilla after it is thickened and add to a Mason jar.

2. It's so easy to combine the smoothie. Just blend, and enjoy

Yields: One serving

Chocolate Cinnamon Smoothie – Keto and Paleo

Ingredients

½ ripened avocado

¾ cup coconut milk

1 teaspoon cinnamon powder

2 teaspoons unsweetened cacao powder

¼ teaspoon vanilla extract

To Taste: Stevia

Optional: 1 teaspoon coconut oil or 1/2 teaspoon MCT Oil

Instructions

1. Blend all of the above ingredients well and enjoy!

Yields: One Serving (Keto)

Chocolate-Covered Strawberries Smoothie - Paleo

Ingredients

½ cup unsweetened strawberries (frozen)

¾ cup (divided) skim milk

12 large ice cubes (divided)

1 pouch rich milk chocolate (no sugar added) - Carnation Breakfast Essentials

Optional: 2 tablespoons water

Instructions

Preparation Layer 1: Place the strawberries on the first layer of the blender, four ice cubes, and ¼ cup of the milk. Pulse until the mixture is creamy smooth. Empty into a glass, and place in the freezer.

Preparation Layer 2: Add the rest of the milk and the breakfast powder into the blender. Pulse until no lumps are remaining. Pour in the ice and pulse again.

Note: Use the water if the combinations are too thick.

Combination: Create your own masterpiece with the alternating layers. The ideas are endless!

Chocolate Raspberry - Vegan

Ingredients

1 cup organic plant milk – ex. fortified rice

1 banana

1 cup baby spinach

2/3 cup frozen raspberries

¼ teaspoon pure vanilla extract

1 tablespoon each:

- Chopped walnuts

- Dark unsweetened cocoa powder

Instructions

1. Add each of the components into a high-speed blender for about 30 seconds.

Yields: One serving

Coconut Cream Pie Smoothie

Ingredients

1 cup 2% milk

Meat from 1 young coconut

½ cup canned coconut milk

1 tablespoon each:

- Meringue powder

- Granulated sugar

1 graham cracker rectangle

¼ teaspoon coconut extract

Instructions

1. Add all of the ingredients into the blender. Crumble an extra cracker on top and enjoy.

Yields: One serving (16 ounces)

Coconut Green Smoothie

Ingredients

½ cup each

- Plain Greek yogurt

- Coconut milk

1 cup spinach

1 large peeled banana

1 large apple (peel, core, and chop)

1 cup ice

2 tablespoons shaved coconut

Instructions

1. Pour the milk, yogurt, and rest of the makings into a blender.

2. Mix until creamy and enjoy.

Yields: One serving

"Up-and-At-'em" Coffee Smoothie

Ingredients

¼ cup coconut milk

2 bananas

½ cup coffee (room temperature or cold)

Optional: 2-3 tablespoons coconut flakes

Handful of ice

Instructions

1. Combine all of the parts in a food processor/blender for about 20 seconds or so.

2. Garnish with a swirl of chocolate or some flaked coconut.

Yields: Two servings

Coffee – Banana Smoothie

Ingredients

½ cup drained silken tofu

1 ¼ - cups low-fat milk

2 teaspoons instant coffee powder – espresso preferred

1 tablespoon sugar/to taste

1 ripe banana

2 ice cubes

Optional: Ground cinnamon

Instructions

1. Combine the ingredients in a blender, mixing until frothy.

2. Taste and add more sweetener if desired. Enjoy with a sprinkle of cinnamon.

Yields: Two servings

Cucumber Ginger Smoothie

Ingredients

1 juiced lemon

1 ½ - cups water

¼ avocado

½ cup cucumber

1 cup baby spinach

2 Medjool dates

½ teaspoon ground ginger

2 tablespoons hemp seeds

2 dashes sea salt

1 cup ice

Instructions

1. Peel and pit the avocado and cucumber. Discard the pits from the dates.

2. Use a high-speed blender using the lowest speed first.

3. Blend about 35 seconds.

Yields: Two servings

Frozen Peppermint Hot Chocolate - Keto

Ingredients

3 ounces – 85% dark chocolate

1 ½-cups unsweetened almond milk

½ cup chocolate protein powder

1 teaspoon peppermint liquid stevia

½ teaspoon peppermint extract

2 cups ice

Instructions

1. Blend each of the ingredients in a high-powered blender.

2. Add sweetener as desired.

Yields: Four (32-ounce) servings

Fruity Easter Egg Smoothie - Paleo

Ingredients

9 (divided) ice cubes

9 tablespoons water (divided)

9 tablespoons non-fat milk (divided)

½ cup each of frozen:

- Blueberries

- Strawberries

- Pineapple

Instructions

1. Duplicate the process for each one.

2. Add 3 Tablespoons of water, 3 Tablespoons of milk, and 3 ice cubes along with the fruit in the blender.

3. Pour each of the prepared ingredients into a glass and place it in the freezer and move on until you finish the three units.

4. To serve, alternate the three tasty glasses into a serving glass/glasses, and enjoy.

Yields: 2 Small or 1 large smoothie

Make as many as you wish and share with your friends and family!

Grape Smoothie

Ingredients

½ cup grape juice

1 cup frozen red – seedless – grapes

¼ cup low-fat plain yogurt

Instructions

1. This one is so easy. Use the blender and pour all of the ingredients into it and process until it's frothy.

Yields: 1 serving (1 ½ cups)

Grasshopper Pie Smoothie

Ingredients

1 cup 2% milk

2 cups fresh spinach

5 fresh mint leaves

¼ teaspoon peppermint extract

2 tablespoons each:

- Granulated sugar

- Cocoa powder

6 ice cubes

Instructions

1. Combine all of the components of the smoothie in a blender for around 30 seconds. Pour and enjoy.

Yields: One serving (16 ounces)

Green Tea – Banana – Blueberry Smoothie

Ingredients

1 green tea bag

3 tablespoons water

¾ cup calcium-fortified light vanilla soy milk

2 teaspoons honey

½ of a medium banana

1 ½ cups frozen blueberries

Instructions

1. Heat the water in the microwave until it boils. Add the bag and brew three minutes. Discard the bag and pour in the honey.

2. Mix the banana, berries, and milk along with the tea to a blender.

3. Use the highest setting until smooth. (You may need a little more water.)

Yields: One serving

Kale and Apple Detox Smoothie

Ingredients

1 chopped celery stalk

1 ½ cups chopped kale

2/3 cup almond milk - unsweetened

1 tbsp. ground flaxseed

½ green/red apple cored and chopped

¾ cup ice

Optional: 1 tsp. honey

Instructions

1. Simply add all of the ingredients into a blender until mixed thoroughly.

Yields: One to two servings

Kale Strawberry Banana Detox Smoothie

Ingredients

1 cup of each:

- Chopped kale

- Plain yogurt

- Strawberries (fresh or frozen)

- Ice

1 banana

Instructions

1. Simply add all of the ingredients into a blender until mixed thoroughly.

Yields: One to two servings

Kale Pineapple Coconut Detox Smoothie

Ingredients

1 banana

1 cup of each:

- Pineapple

- Coconut milk

2 cups chopped kale

Instructions

1. Combine, blend, and enjoy!

Keto Green Smoothie Version 1

The Famous Green Smoothie

Ingredients

2 ripe bananas

3 cups spinach

1 cup coconut/plain water

3 cups frozen fruit

- Peaches

- Pineapple

- Mango

Instructions

1. Blend/puree the entire batch of the additives.

2. Serve or freeze the treat for later.

Yields: Four servings

Keto Green Smoothie – Version 2

Ingredients

1 teaspoon – 1 tablespoon MCT Oil

1 scoop Whey Protein

2 tablespoons each:

- Chia seeds

- Flax meal

2 cups frozen spinach

3 cups water

5 ice cubes

Instructions

1. Blend all of the ingredients on the high setting for 30 seconds until the spinach is almost liquefied.

Note: MCT Oil can be purchased at Wal-Mart. Use one teaspoon of the oil until your body adjusts.

Yields: 1 (Serving is 32 ounces)

Keto Green Smoothie – Version 3

Ingredients

1 cup romaine lettuce

1/3 cup fresh chopped pineapple

4 cups filtered water

2 tablespoons fresh parsley

1 tablespoon fresh ginger

½ cup kiwi fruit

1 cup raw cucumber

½ avocado

1 tablespoon granulated sugar substitute - Swerve

Instructions

1. Blend all of the ingredients until smooth.

Note: You can save leftovers for several days in the refrigerator.

Yields: (6 – 1 cup servings)

Key Lime Pie Smoothie – Paleo

Ingredients

½ avocado

1 cup coconut milk

Zest and juice 2 limes

Honey/sweetener to taste

Instructions

1. Add the avocado, milk, lime, and honey to a blender. Process until it's smooth.

Yields: Two servings

Kiwi-Banana Smoothie

Ingredients

½ cup ice cubes

1- kiwi fruit (1/2 cup)

1 banana

1 cup yogurt (low-fat)

Optional: 2 teaspoons maple syrup

Instructions

1. Peel and cut the Kiwi fruit and banana into chunks.

2. Blend everything on the list until smooth and serve immediately.

Yields: Two Servings

La Isla Bonita

Ingredients

½ cup each:

- Frozen kale

- Coconut water

1 peeled frozen banana

Instructions

1. Blend the entire list of ingredient until smooth.

2. Add a few almonds or ¼ cup of frozen blueberries. For an extra boost add some protein powder.

Yields: One serving

Chapter 3
Leprechaun - Peachy Smoothies

Leprechaun Protein Smoothie - Keto

Ingredients

¼ cup each:

- Coconut milk
- Almond milk/water

1 frozen banana

1/3 cup pumpkin puree

2 cups spinach

¼ teaspoon each:

- Ginger powder
- Cinnamon

4 ice cubes

5 grams whey protein powder

Dash of freshly grated nutmeg

Instructions

1. Peel and cut the banana into chunks

2. Add the yogurt almond milk/water, and coconut milk in a blender. Toss in the remainder of the ingredients

3. Serve with some coconut whipped cream for a special treat.

Yields: One serving

Lime Cantaloupe Smoothie

Ingredients

1/3 cup diced peach

2 cups diced cantaloupe

1 lime

1 tablespoon honey

3 cubes of ice

Instructions

1. Dice the peach and cantaloupe, and grate ½ teaspoon of the lime peel retrieving two tablespoons of the juice.

2. Combine everything until frothy and enjoy.

Yields: One serving (Two cups)

Mango – Apricot – Madness *MAM*

Ingredients

2 ripe mangoes (10-12 ounces each/2 cups)

2 cups/6 apricots

¼ teaspoon vanilla extract

1 cup plain low-fat yogurt/reduced-fat milk

4 teaspoons fresh lemon juice

8 cubes of ice

Garnish: Twists of lemon peel

Instructions

1. Peel and pit the apricots and mangoes.

2. Pour in everything, but the ice, and process in a blender for about eight seconds.

3. Add the ice cubes and continue for about six to eight more seconds until smooth.

Yields: Two servings

Mango Berry Smoothie Bowl - Paleo

Ingredients

¾ cup almond milk

1 ripe (divided) banana

1 cup cubed frozen mango

Options:

- Ground flax seed

- Toasted coconut

- Frozen blueberries

- Frozen raspberries

Instructions

1. Add the milk and ½ of the banana in the blender until smooth.

2. Toss in the mango and –again—blend until creamy smooth.

3. Pour it into your dish and top it off with the optional ingredients of your choice.

Yields: One Serving

Mango Coconut Caribbean Quean

Ingredients

¾ cup (8 pieces) frozen mango

½ cup coconut milk

Instructions

1. Add the milk and mangos into the blender, and mix until smooth.

2. Garnish if desired. With some Garnishes such as protein powder, ground nutmeg, or 2 tablespoons shredded – unsweetened coconut

Yields: One serving

Mango Coconut Green Smoothie

Ingredients

1 cup chopped kale

1/3 cup cottage cheese (low-fat)

½ cup coconut water

1 cup frozen banana slices (1/2 med. banana)

½ cup frozen mango

1 tablespoon flax meal or flaxseed

1-2 teaspoons honey/maple syrup (optional)

Instructions

1. Pour the water and cottage cheese into the blender first. Toss in the remainder of components, and blend until smooth.

Yields: One serving

Mixed Berries and Banana Smoothie

Ingredients

½ c. low-fat frozen yogurt

1 frozen ripe banana

1 c. frozen mixed berries

Optional: 1 teaspoon honey

Instructions

1. Thoroughly blend all of the components and enjoy.

Yields: One to two servings (Two cups)

Monkey Shake Smoothie

Ingredients

1 fully ripe banana

2 cup fat-free milk

1 package (1.4 ounces) fat-free chocolate/sugar-free instant pudding

Last Step: 2 cups crushed ice

Instructions

1. Cut the banana into chunks.

2. Mix all of the listed ingredients (omit the ice) in a blender and mix well.

3. Add the ice, and blend using the high speed until it is creamy smooth.

4. Enjoy it for a super quick breakfast or any other time of the day!

Yields: Four (One - cup servings)

NutriBullet - Smoothie Bowl - Keto

Ingredients

2 tablespoons heavy cream

½ cup almond milk

1 cup spinach

1 scoop low-carb protein powder

1 tablespoon coconut oil

2 ice cubes

Toppings:

4 walnuts

4 raspberries

1 teaspoon chia seeds

1 tablespoon shredded coconut.

Instructions

1. Using a NutriBullet, or a high-speed blender, add the cup of spinach, milk, cream, ice, and coconut oil. Blend it a few seconds until creamy and pour into a bowl.

Be creative if you wish, and add the additional toppings.

Orange Dream Smoothie

Ingredients

¼ cup fat-free yogurt/half and half

¼ teaspoon vanilla extract

1 peeled navel orange

2 tablespoons frozen orange juice concentrate

4 cubes of ice

Instructions

1. Process all of the parts in a high-speed blender about 30 seconds until smooth.

Yields: One serving

Orange Green Ginger Smoothie

Ingredients

1 small banana

1 cup organic rice/plant milk

½ medium peeled orange

1 cup frozen broccoli florets

¼ teaspoon ground ginger

1 tablespoon hemp seeds

Instructions

1. Blend all of the ingredients for approximately 30 seconds in a high-speed blender. Yummy!

Yields: One serving

PB&J Smoothie

Ingredients

1 cup of each:

- Skim milk

- Frozen strawberries

1 banana

¼ cup peanut butter (+) more for garnish if desired

2 tablespoons fresh – chopped – strawberries

Instructions

1. Toss in all of the ingredients into a high-speed blender - until creamy.

Yields: Two servings

Papaya - Strawberry Smoothie

Ingredients

1 cup sliced papaya

½ cup strawberries

1 cup coconut kefir

½ cup ice water

1 scoop vanilla bone broth protein powder or other protein powder of your choice

Instructions

1. Empty all of the parts into a blender and combine until smooth.

Yields: Two servings

Papaya Tropical Smoothie

Ingredients

1 papaya – in chunks

1 cup plain yogurt - fat-free

½ cup each:

- Crushed ice

- Fresh pineapple chunks

1 teaspoon each:

- Ground flaxseed

- Coconut extract

Instructions

1. Mix all of the components in a high-speed blender.

2. Process it for about 30 seconds until frosty and creamy smooth.

Yields: One serving

Peaches and Cream Oatmeal Smoothie

Ingredients

1 cup of each:

- Almond milk

- Unsweetened Greek yogurt

- Frozen peach slices

¼ teaspoon vanilla extract

¼ cup oatmeal

Instructions

1. Add the liquids first followed by all other ingredients and blend until smooth.

Peachy Smoothie Delight

Ingredients

2 tablespoons yogurt -- low-fat vanilla

½ cup each

- Strawberries

- Frozen peaches

2 teaspoons whey protein powder

1/8 teaspoon powdered ginger

1 cup 1% milk

3 cubes of ice

Instructions

1. Blend all of the liquid ingredients and add the whey powder to ensure the grains are evenly distributed.

2. Combine the remainder of the fixings with the ice as the last one. The more volume, the more ice to lower the calories!

Yields: Two servings

Chapter 4

Peanut Butter – Pumpkin Pie Smoothies

Peanut Butter – Banana Cream Pie Smoothie

Ingredients

1 banana

1 cup almond milk

1 teaspoon vanilla extract

2 tablespoons peanut butter

1 rectangle – graham cracker

Instructions

1. Pour the milk, and add the banana, peanut butter, and vanilla into a blender.

2. Garnish with a crumbled graham cracker.

Yields: 1 serving (16 ounces)

Peanut Butter Cup Smoothie

Ingredients

½ cup vanilla frozen yogurt (low-fat)

1 cup of each:

- Ripe sliced banana

- Chocolate 1% low-fat milk

1 carton vanilla low-fat yogurt (8 ounces)

2 tablespoons peanut butter (natural-style)

Instructions

1. Freeze the banana in the freezer for about one hour.

2. Take it out and let it stand for about five minutes.

3. Combine all of the ingredients on the list in a blender and work it until the shake is creamy smooth.

Yields: Three servings (one cup each)

Peanut Butter Kale Smoothie

Ingredients

½ cup rice/plant milk

1 frozen banana

1 cup baby kale

1 tablespoon all-natural peanut butter

Instructions

1. Add all of the ingredients into the blender. Use the high-speed setting for about 30 seconds and enjoy.

Yields: One serving

Piña Colada Smoothie

Ingredients

1 cup of each:

- Frozen pineapple

- Coconut milk

1 chilled banana

1 tablespoon shredded coconut (+) more for garnish

Instructions

1. Place all of the tasty treats in a blender using the highest speed. Process until creamy.

Yields: Two servings

Piña Colada - Chia Seed Smoothie

Ingredients

½ cup unsweetened/coconut Greek yogurt

1 tablespoon Chia seeds

1 cup each:

- Coconut milk

- Frozen pineapple chunks

- 1 teaspoon flaked coconut

Optional:

- 1 teaspoon coconut oil

- 1 lime wedge – garnish

Instructions

1. You know the drill. Combine, blend, and serve.

Yields: One serving

Pineapple Mojito Smoothie

Ingredients

¼ cup fresh mint

3 cups chopped pineapple

1 juiced lime

2 cups each:

- Coconut Unsweetened water

- Kale/spinach with stems removed

Instructions

1. Blend the mint, kale, and chosen water until creamy.

2. Add the lime juice, and pineapple, blending until smooth. Woo Hoo!

Yields: Two servings

Pineapple Passion Smoothie

Ingredients

1 cup pineapple chunks

6 ice cubes

1 cup light/low-fat vanilla yogurt

Instructions

1. Mix the ice cubes with the yogurt. Blend and pulse until it has large chunks.

2. Add the chunks of pineapple and process on the highest setting until smooth.

Yields: One serving

Pomegranate – Banana Smoothie

Ingredients

2 cups pure pomegranate juice

2 large bananas

2 cups non-fat plain yogurt

Instructions

1. Blend the juice with the yogurt and add the sliced bananas—puree.

Note: the pomegranate can be bottled or fresh squeezed.

Yields: Six servings

Pumpkin – Apple Smoothie

Ingredients

¾ cup Greek yogurt

¼ cup canned pumpkin

¼ cup (+) 2 tablespoons old-fashioned oats

1 medium apple

Instructions

1. Slice the apple and banana into pieces.

2. Toss the oats in a blender for 30 seconds, and add the remainder of the ingredients. Process it until it's creamy.

Yields: Two servings

Pumpkin – Pecan Pie Smoothie

Ingredients

¾ cup pumpkin puree

1 cup 2% milk

½ cup plain low-fat yogurt

¼ cup toasted pecans

1 teaspoon ground cinnamon

2 tablespoons maple syrup

¼ teaspoon ground cloves

½ teaspoon ground ginger

Instructions

1. Add each of the fixings into a blender and continue on the highest setting until the nuts are smooth and combined.

Yields: One serving (16 ounces)

Pumpkin Pie Smoothie

Ingredients

½ cup each:

- Vanilla soy milk

- Canned pumpkin

- Crushed ice

1 teaspoon pumpkin pie spice

1 tablespoon honey

Instructions

1. Combine all of the ingredients in a blender for about 20-30 seconds and serve.

2. Be festive!

Yields: One serving

Pumpkin Pie Spice Mango Smoothie

Ingredients

1 cup rice milk

1 Medjool date– pitted

¼ cup frozen cut leaf spinach/½ cup baby spinach

½ cup frozen mango chunks

½ teaspoon pumpkin pie spice

1 tablespoon chia seeds

Instructions

1. Toss the ingredients into your blender on the slowest setting, increasing to the highest speed by 40 seconds. Pour and enjoy right away.

Yields: One serving

Chapter 5
Raspberry - Strawberry Smoothies

Raspberry Delight

Ingredients

2 very ripe bananas

½ cup plain yogurt

1 cup of each:

- Fresh spinach

- Frozen raspberries

- Coconut/plain water

Instructions

1. Blend each of the ingredients until smooth and serve cold. So tasty!

Yields: Two servings

Raspberry Avocado Smoothie - Keto

Ingredients

3 tablespoons lemon juice

1 1/3 cup water

1 ripe avocado

½ cup frozen unsweetened raspberries/or choice of berries

1 tablespoon (+) 1 teaspoon sugar equivalent

Instructions

1. Blend all of the components in a blender until creamy smooth.

2. Empty the smoothie into two chilled glasses and enjoy!

Yields: Two servings

Red Velvet Smoothie

Ingredients

4 medium hulled fresh/frozen strawberries

¾ cup chopped/grated raw red beets

1 frozen banana

2 dried – pitted – sliced dates

1 cup skim/almond milk (unsweetened)

1 tbsp. agave syrup

2 tbsp. cocoa powder

Instructions

1. Blend it all together and enjoy

Yields: Two cups

Rosemary Mango Smoothie

Ingredients

1 banana

½ lime – juiced

1 cup rice milk

½ cup baby spinach

1 cup frozen chopped mango

¼ teaspoon ground ginger

1 tablespoon each:

- Raw pumpkin seeds
- Fresh rosemary

Instructions

1. Mix all of the fixings in a blender using the high setting for about 35 seconds. Enjoy!

Yields: One serving

Soy Mania Smoothie

Ingredients

1 sliced frozen banana

1 cup calcium-fortified vanilla soy milk

½ cup each:

- Cornflakes cereal

- Frozen blueberries

Instructions

1. Combine the banana, milk, corn flakes, and berries for 20 seconds in a blender.

2. Scrape the sides and blend for another 15 seconds until it is well mixed.

Yields: One serving

Spicy-Sweet Green Pea Smoothie

Ingredients

1 cup natural tomato juice – no salt

4 baby carrots

½ cup frozen peas

2 pitted Medjool dates

1 chopped celery stalk

1/8 teaspoon each:

- Fine sea salt

- Cayenne pepper

Instructions

1. Using a high-speed blender at the lowest speed, combine all of the ingredients. Work up to the highest speed for 35 seconds and serve immediately.

Yields: One serving

Strawberry Almond Banana Smoothie

Ingredients

¼ cup plain low-fat yogurt

½ cup frozen strawberries

1 frozen peeled banana

1 cup water

Pinch of salt

1 tablespoon each:

- Honey

- Almond butter (or adjust to taste)

Instructions

1. Empty all of the ingredients in the blender. Process for about 30 seconds, and sprinkle with some salt.

Yields: One serving

Strawberry Banana Frozen Smoothie

Ingredients

2 cups frozen strawberries/cherries

1 cup milk

½ cup each:

- Freshly squeezed orange juice

- Vanilla/plain yogurt

1 frozen banana

2 to 3 tablespoons honey

Instructions

1. Blend all of the makings until creamy.

Note: if you want a non-dairy smoothie, substitute one cup of rice milk for the yogurt and milk. You can also use soy yogurt or milk.

Yields: Two servings

Strawberry Banana Frozen Smoothie Version 2

Ingredients

1 cup fresh strawberries

2 cups chopped kale

1 medium banana

½ cup skim milk

1 cup ice cubes

Optional: 1 to 2 tablespoons honey

Instructions

1. Mix all of the ingredients in a blender and mix for about 30 seconds or until it's creamy smooth.

Yields: One serving

Strawberry Broccoli Coconut Surprise Smoothie

Ingredients

1 ripened banana

1 cup of each:

- Frozen broccoli florets
- Almond milk
- Frozen sliced strawberries

2 tablespoons each:

- Unsweetened shredded coconut
- Hemp seeds

1 pitted Medjool date

¼ teaspoon cinnamon

½ teaspoon pure vanilla extract

Instructions

1. Dump all of the ingredients into a high-speed blender and puree for about 30 seconds. Enjoy!

Yields: One smoothie

Strawberry –Kiwi Smoothie

Ingredients

1 sliced kiwi

1 ripe sliced banana

1 ¼ cup cold apple juice

5 frozen strawberries

1 ½ teaspoons honey

Instructions

1. Blend it all until smooth and creamy. What a treat!

Yields: Four servings

Strawberry-Oatmeal Smoothie

Ingredients

2 scoops protein powder (unsweetened/30 g protein per scoop)

½ cup instant oatmeal

1 cup frozen strawberries

1 medium banana

1 ½ cups skim milk

Optional: ¼ teaspoon vanilla

Instructions

1. Use a blender to combine all of the ingredients until creamy smooth.

2. Refrigerate or serve right away.

Yields: Four Servings

Strawberry Banana Pineapple Smoothie

Ingredients

1 medium banana

½ cup each:

- Fresh strawberries

- Cubed fresh pineapple

¼ cup each:

- Fresh pineapple juice

- Skim milk

Optional: 1 cup ice cubes

Instructions

1. Dump all of the goodies in a blender and mix until creamy - about 30 seconds.

Yields: One serving

Strawberry Shortcake Smoothie - Paleo

Ingredients

¾ cup non-dairy or non-fat milk

1 cup unsweetened frozen strawberries

1 teaspoon butter extract

Optional: Sweetener to taste

Instructions

1. Use a blender and combine everything on the list; beginning with:

   - Strawberries

   - Milk

   - Butter extract

2. Serve and totally enjoy!

Yields: One serving

Strawberry Swing

Ingredients

8 frozen strawberries

½ cup each:

- Pourable plain yogurt/plain kefir

- Unsweetened – shredded coconut

Instructions

1. Add each of the components of this healthy choice into a blender.

2. Process until well blended.

3. *For some Changes:* Add 2 tablespoons rolled oats, 2 tablespoons flax meal, some protein powder, or a pinch of ground cinnamon.

Yields: One serving

Strawberry Swiss Chard Smoothie

Ingredients

1 cup plant milk (ex. rice milk)

1 small banana

3-4 leaves Swiss chard

1 tablespoon each:

Sliced almonds

Shredded unsweetened coconut

½ cup frozen strawberries

Instructions

1. Remove the leaves from the chard, and slice the strawberries.

2. Add the ingredients to a blender starting with its lowest speed for about 30 seconds.

Yields: One serving

Chapter 6
Sunrise - Watermelon Smoothies

Sunrise Smoothie

Ingredients

1 container low-fat vanilla yogurt

1 small banana

1 cup each:

- Whole strawberries

- Ice

4 ounces low-calorie orange soda

Note: Sunkist is a good choice.

Instructions

1. Cut the banana into chunks.

2. Add the yogurt to the blender—followed by the banana—blending until smooth.

3. Add the soda—blend—then the ice—and blend until creamy smooth.

Yields: Two Servings

Sweet Potato Pie Smoothie

Ingredients

1 ½ cups fortified rice milk/your choice of plant milk

1 cup frozen broccoli florets

1 sweet potato

2 Medjool dates – pitted

½ tablespoon chia seeds

½ teaspoon pumpkin pie spice

Instructions

1. Bake the sweet potato and remove the skin.

2. Toss all of the ingredients into a blender on the high speed for 30 seconds.

Yields: Five servings

Tutti-Frutti Smoothie

Ingredients

½ cup each:

- Orange juice

- Sliced ripened banana

- Mixed frozen berries/strawberries

- Plain yogurt

- Canned - crushed pineapple – in juice

Instructions

1. You can use an immersion blender in a large measuring cup.

2. Or, use the food processor fitted with a metal blade.

3. Or, use the trusty blender to combine all ingredients until creamy smooth.

Yields: Two servings

Vanilla Smoothie - Keto

Ingredients

2 large egg yolks

¼ cup water

½ cup mascarpone full-fat cheese

½ teaspoon pure vanilla extract

4 ice cubes

1 tablespoon each:

- Powdered Erythritol /3 drops liquid Stevia

- Coconut oil

Optional: Whipped cream

Instructions

1. Mix all of the components into a blender and pulse until creamy smooth.

2. Provide your choice of garnishes.

Yields: One serving

Vegan Breakfast Smoothie

Ingredients

1 small banana

1 c. rice/almond milk

1 c. fresh dark green leafy veggie – ex. Kale or spinach

1 c. frozen fruit – ex. Pineapple or blueberries

1 tablespoon seeds or nuts – ex. Pumpkin, flax, or hemp

1-2 tablespoons Medjool dates – pitted/1-2 tablespoons shredded coconut

Instructions

1. Combine everything in a high-speed blender for 30 seconds. (Begin slowly and increase the speed.)

Yields: One serving

Vegan Fruit Smoothie

Ingredients

½ cup peaches/frozen berries

¼ cup silken tofu

¾ cup orange juice

Honey or sugar if desired

Instructions

1. Add the ingredients to a blender and combine until smooth.

Yields: One serving

Watermelon Berry Smoothie – Paleo

Ingredients

1 cup frozen blueberries

2 cups watermelon - cubed

1 cup fresh raspberries

1 – ½ cups ice

Instructions

1. In a high-speed blender, combine all of the ingredients until smooth.

Watermelon Enchantment Smoothie

Ingredients

¼ cup fat-free milk

2 cups Chopped watermelon

Ice (approx. 2 cups)

Instructions

1. Blend the milk and watermelon for about 15 seconds, until smooth.

2. Pour on the ice and continue mixing for about 20 seconds.

Yields: Two servings

Watermelon Rehydration Smoothie

Ingredients

½ cup coconut water

1 cup watermelon chunks

4 mint leaves

1 ½ teaspoon lime juice

4 ice cubes

Instructions

1. Mix all of the fixings in a blender for 20-30 seconds until smooth.

Yields: One serving

Conclusion

Thank you for making it through to the end of *Ketogenic Diet for Beginners: 4-Week Plan for Weight Loss*. Let's hope it was informative and provided you with all of the tools you need to achieve your goals with these tasty smoothies, whatever they may be.

The next step is to go to the market or just look in your fridge to see what you need to get going. The ingredients are all tested to ensure they are of the highest quality. You will know once you have them in your blender.